THE PRICELESS GIFT SURVIVING CANCER

YMA ORNÉ CAMPBELL

authorHOUSE®

AuthorHouse™
1663 Liberty Drive
Bloomington, IN 47403
www.authorhouse.com
Phone: 1 (800) 839-8640

Published by AuthorHouse   09/23/2016

ISBN: 978-1-5246-4143-6 (sc)
ISBN: 978-1-5246-4142-9 (e)

Print information available on the last page.

This book is printed on acid-free paper.

THE HOLY BIBLE, NEW INTERNATIONAL VERSION®, NIV® Copyright © 1973,
1978, 1984, 2011 by Biblica, Inc.® Used by permission. All rights reserved worldwide.

Jeremiah 29:11
New International Version (NIV)

11 For I know the plans I have for you," declares the Lord, "plans to prosper you and not to harm you, plans to give you hope and a future.

DEDICATIONS

This book is dedicated to everyone! It is a memory for those who have battled cancer and lost and reminder for those who have fought cancer and won! It is hope for those who are still fighting and will continue to fight, please don't give up...I am with you, I am for you, and I am praying...I love you

1

I'M SORRY, IT'S CANCER...

It was Tuesday afternoon May 17th, a beautiful day in North Carolina and my second son's (Khalief) 22nd birthday. I was so excited because I was thinking about making him a cake. I know that he loves cake and he likes to keep it simple. I even thought about getting some Spanish food from one of our favorite restaurants. As I think back I don't remember what we did because the next few hours after 2pm are still a blur. My mind went and never returned to the joy that I felt for my second son.

My oldest son (Keith) and I were at Duke Hospital in Durham, North Carolina. I had taken the morning off from work because I wanted to get these results from the doctor so that I could return to my everyday life. I had gone to another doctor prior who had told me that he didn't know for sure what the problem was. My oldest son and I sat quietly in the cold room waiting patiently for the doctor. That was the longest wait. I remained positive although I was worried. I kept happy thoughts in my mind. I prayed and meditated. I even found peace in playing with my cell phone. I was not prepared for what would happen next.

The doctor came in and she firmly shook my hand. She was very friendly and presented with a warm and caring demeanor. She had her folder in her hand with my results. She knew that I had a biopsy prior to coming to her office for the visit. She sat down and looked at me and asked me what the other doctor told me. I told her that the other told me that he was not sure if it was cancer but. She stopped me in the middle of my sentence and said its cancer. I sat in the exam chair and my mouth dropped open. I was in shock. The doctor looked at me and said, "I am so sorry. You have Papillary Thyroid Cancer." I began to weep and cry. It seemed as if my whole life had passed before my eyes. For a moment I went into a deep thought as I began to think about my family. I began to asked questions that only God could answer. I asked what would happen to everyone without me. Where would they go? Where would they be? The pain had begun to intensify because those words, you have cancer, had already started to pierce my heart. My oldest son was with me. He is a current medical student and told and whispered to me, "Mom you are going to be ok." The doctor handed me some tissue as the tears rolled down my cheeks. All of my dreams seemed to stop in the process. Everything that I wanted was not of importance at this moment. The only thing I could ask for at this point was for life. I just wanted to live.

After I had my moment to process, I realize that there would be other moments. This roller coaster of emotions was just beginning. My doctor had told me that she was going to set me up with appointments. She discussed the cancer as if it was a plan to attack. She assured me that we would beat this and we would not leave any stone unturned. I had another issue that was very concerning in addition to the cancer; I was diagnosed with Primary Hyperparathyroidism Disease resulting from an elevated PTH (parathyroid hormone test). In other words, my blood calcium levels were higher than normal and that meant that I had a parathyroid that was malfunctioning in my body. As a result of the malfunctioning parathyroid I was experiencing symptoms of muscle weakness, lethargy, and fatigue, pain in my muscles (burning sensation in my legs), depression, frequent urination, nausea, impaired memory, personality changes, and constipation.

I needed more of an explanation. I couldn't understand how I could have been so healthy, had good physicals annually and suddenly to be impacted with a cancer diagnosis and now Hyperparathyroidism Disease. My doctor gave me some information and explained it to me in manner that I could understand. She even provided me with a drawing and pointed out the position of the thyroid and the location of the parathyroid. I understood it that the parathyroid glands are four small glands located near or on the back of the thyroid gland. They produce parathyroid hormone (PTH). Parathyroid glands are normally very small. They are generally about the size of a single grain of rice. However, sometimes one or more becomes enlarged. It then produces too much PTH. In other cases, a growth on one of these glands can cause increased PTH. An increased amount of PTH leads to too much calcium in your blood. Primary hyperparathyroidism occurs when your parathyroid glands produce too much PTH. This can happen if you have an adenoma (a benign tumor of glandular tissue) or non-cancerous tumor on one of these glands. These tumors are the most common cause of primary hyperparathyroidism.

The discussion overall addressed the Papillary Thyroid Cancer and the Primary Hyperparathyroidism Disease as these were both two problems that were beginning to be a problem for me and my body and could be potentially life threatening if not addressed in a timely manner. I was informed that surgery was definitely necessary to address these issues. She had me scheduled for a lymph node mapping (an ultrasound done to look and see if the cancer has spread beyond the site of the thyroid). I was also scheduled for a Nuclear Medicine Sestamibi Scan (Parathyroid Scan). The purpose of the Nuclear Medicine Sestamibi Scan is to detect parathyroid adenomas (tumors) in patients with sporadic primary hyperparathyroidism. The Nuclear Medicine Sestamibi scanning will never show a normal parathyroid gland.

My appointments were scheduled and my surgery was scheduled for June 6th. I had a birthday coming up toward the end of the month and I promised myself that I was going to enjoy it. I thanked my doctor and told her that I looked forward to seeing her on June 6th. I shook her hand and I told her that I trust her expertise and her recommendations. She smiled as she walked out of the exam room.

I was overwhelmed with information. The initial shock was over and I was on my way to work. I didn't have much of an afternoon left because the day was almost over. I returned to work but it was not work as usual. I remember driving and thinking about the fact that I have cancer. My whole life will change. My existence will be important. The things that I took for granted have become important to me. I have to apologize to myself for not loving myself enough to keep up with the things that matter most, my health.

I returned home later that evening and got on the phone and made calls and sent text messages. I told everyone in my family and some of my very close friends that the news is what I dreaded the most, cancer. I had to tell everyone I was diagnosed with thyroid cancer. I felt horrible because I couldn't celebrate my son's 22nd birthday the way I normally would. I was saddened by the thought that I may have missed out on a celebration and not knowing if it were my last. I cried hysterically as I walked off alone to myself. My husband had a look of grief and overwhelming sadness. He held me and told me that we would get through this and cancer was not going to rent any space in our home or our minds. I received numerous words of encouragement and support. I was most appreciative of everyone but the most heart wrenching thing for me was that I had to live my life as if it was hanging in the balance. I had a fear of the unknown. There is one thing that was certain for me and that was that today was almost over, yesterday was gone, and tomorrow was not promised.

Philippians 4:6-7
New International Version (NIV)

6 Do not be anxious about anything, but in every situation, by prayer and petition, with thanksgiving, present your requests to God. 7 And the peace of God, which transcends all understanding, will guard your hearts and your minds in Christ Jesus.

2

PLEADING WITH GOD

I remember waking up the next morning thinking that it was all a bad dream. I was so exhausted. I couldn't focus on anything else because the thoughts of the cancer had begun to consume me daily. I recall crying daily and thinking about how short life really is. I always remember hearing people say that life is so short but I really had a chance to really think about that statement. I remember praying and crying and talking with God extensively. Am I going to die? What have I done? Why me? Please God, I kept thinking and praying to myself. I cried until my eyes were swollen. I then began to bargain with God as I pleaded with God for my life. I remember praying and telling God how much I do for others. I told God that I was a social worker and I believed that all people deserve a chance even those that do the most harm. I couldn't keep crying and worrying because it wasn't getting me anywhere. I then thought for a moment that if I embrace the sickness then I could advocate for myself and others. That was an unrealistic thought because I was allowing myself to give into my feelings and emotions. My husband always said to me, "You do not have cancer!" He always lovingly reminded me that God is always in control. He promised and planned a wonderful birthday for me. He always keeps his promises and delivered on that promise too! There was not a day that went by that I didn't think about my illness. I prayed and cried. I also found myself being happy at times when I thought I wouldn't be or shouldn't be.

One morning I decided to attack my mind and my thoughts. I told myself that I wasn't going to feel sorry for myself. I said my prayers and did some research. I found non-profit organizations online that provided a wealth of free information. I began to feel connected to people that I didn't even know. I joined two groups on social media where I bonded instantly with people that had gone through some of the same medical issues that I was dealing with. I read their stories and exchanged mine. I felt encouraged and empowered because the more I knew the better I could be to myself and others.

I finally realized in the midst of my crying and depression that all I need to do was to share. It was fine for me to plead with God but it was then that I realized that God wanted me to do more than plead, this is where the strength came in. It was time for me to turn this into something greater that could not only benefit me but benefit others and those around me. It was at that point that I decided that I needed to share. Sharing is such an important part of who we are and how we grow. People that don't share accept themselves at one level and become complacent. They are not open and most times do not know how to open up themselves to anyone especially if they can't be open and honest with themselves.

I decided that I was going to Share. It was against what I was used to. I always thought that it was best to keep things to myself. I thought that sharing personal information about myself with others would only place me in a bad position for people to talk about me and frown upon me negatively. I had to escape that mindset. The support groups on social media gave me the biggest strength because people willingly shared and answered the questions of strangers to help others as they journey through their illness.

On May 20th I decided to publically post on social media that I was diagnosed with cancer. My post is as follows:

It is with a heavy heart that I inform my Facebook family and friends that on Tuesday 5/17/16, I learned that I have Thyroid Cancer (Papillary Cancer). I was in a car accident two years ago on 12/19/14 in which I was T-boned on my side of the car. God was with me and it is that accident that saved my life. A CT-Scan revealed that I had three nodules on my Para-Thyroid. I allowed time to go by but eventually followed up on it when God placed on my heart for me to do so. After three ultra-sounds, a Fine Needle Biopsy and several doctor's appointments, I learned that I have a condition called Hyperparathyroidism and a new nodule located on my Thyroid which is cancerous. I am sharing this with you to create awareness. I appreciate your prayers, and support. Please know your numbers. Listen to your body and know the signs. Everyone should have an annual check-up to know where they stand. I want to now take this opportunity and thank each and every one of you who have made a commitment to pray for me. I genuinely appreciate it very much. I am scheduled to have surgery next month in two weeks. I trust God and believe that

God will heal me. However realizing that life is so incredibly short, I just want to express how much I love you all. During the course of my journey, I have met some of the most wonderful people. I have made friendships that will forever be etched in my heart. My life is a rainbow of love and laughter. Thank you all so much for adding to the Joy that I have experienced. If you are on my Facebook page it is because you mean a lot to me as a person, a friend and my family! I will keep you all posted and again, please keep the prayers going for me.

With much love and blessings…Yma

After my post I felt a sense of freedom. The weight and the burden of my pain and the illness had been lifted. I didn't have to burden God because He knew already. However I did share the weight with others because I wanted them to join me in my crusade to believe God for healing. It was within moments after my post, people began to call, respond to my post, text, and pray. I was blessed beyond measure to have such wonderful people in my life that genuinely cared. The responses were overwhelming and helped me get through the most difficult phases in the weeks ahead. I am so glad that I decided to share. My sharing helped me and allowed me to help others. I was able to learn and did some research of my own. I was able to better understand what I was going through and how it had impacted me so much. I shared my lessons with others. In all of my sharing, I learned and realized that other people were dealing with the same problems and some of their problems were worse than mine.

On Tuesday May 24th, one week after my cancer diagnosis and two days before my birthday, the reality of what was happening and going on had become real for me. I went to have all of my testing done. I had the lymph node mapping to check to see if the cancer has spread and then I had the Nuclear Medicine Sestamibi scan. This was an all-day procedure. I went to the cancer center. I had to spend the entire day there. I had the lymph node mapping and then I had to wait an hour and have the scan completed. I had lunch and then walked around to allow time to pass by. I can recall looking at the many different faces as I walked through the cancer center. Cancer does not have a specific age, race, religion, color, or gender. It can happen to anyone at any time in their life when they least suspect and are not thinking about it or anticipating the worse. The décor in the cancer center was beautiful. The walls were golden in color and the cancer center had a gift shop that had so many beautiful reminders and t-shirts for everyone that wants to show their support for those with cancer. I sat in a chair comfortably outside the gift shop and watched people walked by to the elevators and from the elevators. I watched people walk in and out of the gift shop. Some people purchased wigs, some purchased scarfs, and other just glanced and walked out. In the background on the lower level was a volunteer playing the piano. It was the instrumental version of some beautiful songs. I can't recall the names of the songs but I do recall sitting and sinking into my chair and crying. I cried while I listened and then I began to pray. I prayed and prayed because I had begun to feel weak mentally and I didn't know how much more I could take. I was ready for this to be over with but fear had begun to settle in my spirit. I had a table and began to write and pray. I found myself pleading with God again:

Dear God:

It is just me again. I am coming to you with a humble heart like that of a child. I don't know what the future holds for me but I do know that presently I am hurting. I hurt because tomorrow is a mystery to me. I hurt because I am not ready for you to close the book on my chapter in this existence. God I want you to know that so many people needs me; my husband, my children, and my parents. And God, I have begun a great work that is currently incomplete. Would you really take me away from all of this now? Oh God please know that this is not a good time so I hope it is not your time. God I have a loving husband with whom my life has just begun; and my parents they need me now more than ever before, they are getting older and their work to help others is taking off in a great direction, and finally God, there is my children. I have four beautiful children who have purpose and promise. I am asking you, begging you, and pleading with you to please allow me to see them walk across the stage when they graduate from college. I don't ask for much. I am only asking for this. I realize that this may even be a bit much to ask since you have always been here for me and given me and provided for me. I acknowledged that you have made a way out of no way when I didn't think that there was even a way to be made. Please God. If it is me who you want to do your work and do something different, then please let me know. It is in Jesus name I pray…Amen.

I wiped my eyes and my face. It was time for my second appointment. I went upstairs to the Nuclear Medicine Department for my Sestimibi Parathyroid Scan. I felt a sense of peace. The sestimibi parathyroid scan is a very useful tool to find the enlarged parathyroid(s) in preparation for surgery to treat the Hyperparathyroidism. The scan was performed in Nuclear Medicine and it took about two hours. First, an injection of radioactive dye is given in my arm. Then Nuclear Medicine Technologist took a picture of my neck region. I had to come out of the machine and wait about 90 minutes. After waiting, additional pictures were taken. There was no pain during the exam, but I had an intravenous catheter (IV) in place. I drank lots of water to flush the metallic taste of the medicine from my mouth.

I was emotionally drained at the end of that day. The tests were not bad but just preparing for the unknown and waiting and watching others. It all had an impact on my mind. My problems are not as bad as I may think that they are. I saw people that had their heads draped in beautiful scarfs in 90 degree weather. They were draped in scarfs to cover their heads after losing hair. I saw other people walking through with a look of courage and strength. They didn't seem to be bothered and their look was one of what appeared to be confident and bold. I was weak but praying to God for strength and peace. It was now a time that I realized that I have to live each day as if it were my last. I couldn't take anything for granted. I also realized that I can't put off for tomorrow what I can do today. There is no better time than the present. My birthday was rapidly approaching and my only focus was to celebrate.

Psalm 121:1-2
New International Version (NIV)

1 I lift up my eyes to the mountains; where does my help come from? 2 My help comes from the Lord, the Maker of heaven and earth.

3

THE ACCIDENT THAT SAVED MY LIFE

I can only imagine that if you read this book up to this point, you have a lot of questions for me. One of the main questions that you are probably asking and wondering is; *how did you know you were sick? What or when did you find out? Was this all of a sudden? Why now? Couldn't you have done something sooner?* I am going to answer all of these questions. I hope that after reading this chapter, you will understand how important it is to take your own health seriously and not delay.

It was Friday afternoon on December 19th 2014. I had left work for an extended lunch break because I was scheduled to work late that evening. I decided that I would take my daughter to work and go on back to work. I went home and picked up my daughter. I then stopped at the gas station to get some gas prior to taking her to work. As I was exiting the gas station, I was t-boned on the driver's side of the vehicle. It all happened so fast that I didn't even realize that the air bags had deployed. I was smacked so hard in the face causing a concussion. My daughter was screaming and crying and told me that we were hit. I could not believe that we had been hit. I was in a complete daze. The glass had shattered and I was pinned in on my side of the car. A gentleman came from behind and told me that he saw the whole thing. He told me that help was on the way. I thanked him and asked him to please stay with me until the paramedics arrived. My accident had traffic congested in both ways on the two-lane highway. The paramedics arrived and I asked them to get my daughter out of the car first. We were both transported to the hospital by the paramedics.

Upon our arrival at the hospital, we were both taken into separate rooms and assessed for fractures while tests and other x-rays were ordered. Several hours had passed and the good news is that neither one of us had any broken bones. I had a concussion and would have headaches for several days following the accident. We were discharged to home. As I was getting dressed, the doctor told me that I needed to follow up with my primary care doctor. The doctor stated that I had three small nodules on my neck and they were found during the CAT scan. I asked the doctor was that anything that I really needed to be concerned about. The doctor told me that there was no reason for me to worry about the nodules at that moment but careful follow up should be done to assess the situation to ensure that nothing else is going on. My focus was getting better and getting back to work. It was out of sight and out of mind. The nodules did not bother me and there was no reason for me to bother them. I didn't feel any lumps in my neck and had never been diagnosed with any thyroid problems.

I allowed time to pass maybe longer than I should have. I recovered from my accident and didn't think any more about the nodules in my neck. The holidays had come and gone and a new year was upon us. There was no reason to be concern. My throat was not tight and my voice was not hoarse. I went for my annual physical in early 2015 and my primary care physician called me and told me that I needed to come back in for repeat blood work. I asked her if everything was ok and she told me that my calcium levels were elevated. She further stated that she might have to refer me to an Endocrinologist but wanted to do some more blood work before making that determination. I mentioned the car accident to her and the results of the CAT scan. There didn't sound like any cause for concern in her voice. I returned several days later for the repeat blood work. I received another phone call and this was a voicemail message asking me to call the doctor's office. I never called the doctor's office back. I thought to myself that if I have elevated calcium then I never have to worry about not having enough calcium. I wasn't interested in what elevated calcium means or how it could potentially affect my body or even my life. I was feeling fine for the moment and that is all that mattered to me. I was feeling fine, really. I didn't have any symptoms so I had the thought of; if it's not broke then don't fix it. Therefore I did absolutely nothing.

I decided to allow even more time to pass without doing anything. I do recall as I look back and reflect on it that I was so exhausted. I couldn't understand why I was always so sleepy. I would go to bed tired and wake up tired. I would even go to bed early and still wake up tired. I was so out of it that I didn't even realize that something else could be going on within my body. I kept telling myself that the nodules were nothing. I grabbed my computer and searched the internet and was relieved to know that some people have issues with a goiter, and nodules and there is nothing going on. These people only need to be monitored. I called my mother and she assured me that everything would be fine. My mother told me to pray. She told me that she would be praying but suggested that I get it checked out. I felt a sense of relief but thought about it and came up with the conclusion that it wouldn't hurt for me to go and see the doctor. I searched for an Endocrinologist and found a local one that would be able to evaluate me. I made an appointment and went to be evaluated. They did some blood tests to check my thyroid hormone levels and my parathyroid hormone levels. They also did an ultrasound and saw the three nodules located on my thyroid. There was no cause for concern. I was good with the exam and rescheduled for three months for a follow up. I went back for my follow up and was told that my blood calcium levels were high and that they were going to monitor the levels every three months. I was told that based on the results of the ultrasound that I didn't have anything to worry about. The nodules were very small and there was no reason to be concerned about them at this time. I felt relieved. I followed up like I was supposed to and everything was good. I decided not to go back in three months after because I was feeling good. I thought to myself, except for being tired all the time, there is nothing wrong. After all, the nature of my work causes me to work extremely long hours at time, eat on the go, and have little time to do what I need to do for me. I just didn't have the time or was willing to take the time away from work. My work and cases would pile up if I took some time off. I decided to keep going. I just chose to ignore all of the signs.

The symptoms began to get even more intense. My work load increased or maybe I just couldn't keep up. I was always so tired and exhausted all the time. I would sit down in a chair and immediately fall asleep. I would always feel nauseated for no reason. I then noticed that I could not go to the bathroom. I was always so constipated that I had to take laxatives in order to have a bowel movement. I always felt bloated. I could shake off the tired feeling. I purchased vitamins thinking that they would give me some energy. The vitamins helped for a little while, just enough for me to ignore the signs longer. I also started to feel a little forgetful. My memory and mind was cloudy. I would work on a project and know that I had to do something else to finish and forget totally what was needed to complete it. I decided that it was time to go back to the Endocrinologist and follow up with blood tests to ensure that everything is good. I scheduled an appointment for the early part of the New Year. I managed to get through the holidays without falling part. I had adapted to being tired all the time. I just went along with my body. I allowed my body to be in control. I began to move in accordance to my body. I no longer controlled my movements and my thoughts. I was so exhausted to a point where I didn't think. Everything had become such a routine for me; I had begun to function like a robot. I knew I had to go to work so I would get up and out each day and moved with no thought to how I was feeling. I went to work daily feeling lousy and drained. I would find myself drifting off to sleep if I had to sit in one spot for a long time. I felt like I had to be on the go constantly because if not, I would fall asleep. But when I did fall asleep, I slept like a baby. I could sleep for hours at a time. I recall several times coming home from work and going to bed early. I would get in the bed at 7pm and awaken the next morning at 8 am and I would still be exhausted and drained. There were times that I had to drag myself out of the bed and into work. I kept going and going until it was time to see the doctor. I couldn't go on because my body was beginning the process of breaking down.

I kept my scheduled appointment as planned. I had an ultrasound of my neck. The ultrasound was painless but there were nodules discovered around my thyroid on my parathyroid. I was told that the parathyroid had to be removed at some point but there was no need to worry. The doctor told me that he would just watch the nodules on my parathyroid and keep checking my calcium levels. He further scheduled an appointment for me to return in three months for another ultrasound.

Time passed and I returned for the ultrasound. The ultrasound was painless as it was the last time but this time I was informed that I had to have a biopsy because they saw two nodules on my thyroid. The Endocrinologist told me that the biopsy will let them know if I have cancer. I thought to myself, it can't be, not me. I would not accept cancer and I will not claim such a diagnosis for myself. I am healthy. I kept telling myself that I was healthy and there was nothing wrong with me. I returned within two weeks for the biopsy. It was the most painful procedure that I had to endure. I remember lying on the examination table while the ultrasound tech rubbed the probe on the left side of my neck. Suddenly the doctor stuck a long needle into the left side of my neck. It was painful. I cried as I held my breath. I had my ear buds in my ear as I listened to my husband comforting me. Once the procedure was over the doctor assured me that he would be in touch with me as soon as the results came back. I left his office with the feeling that no news is good news but I will wait patiently. The parathyroid was still there and will have to be removed pending the results from the biopsy.

Several weeks had passed and I didn't hear anything. I called and waited. Then I waited and called. I then contacted the Lab to follow up. The Lab was not able to provide me with any results. I waited and waited some more. I began to think that there could not be anything wrong with me. I felt a sense of relief. I thought to myself that if there was anything wrong I would have known by now.

Isaiah 54:11
New International Version (NIV)

11 Afflicted city, lashed by storms and not comforted,
I will rebuild you with stones of turquoise,
your foundations with lapis lazuli.

4

BRACING FOR THE STORM

It was a Friday afternoon and I was at work. I was the last person in the office and desperately working to finish up a report. My cell phone rang and I answered. It was my Endocrinologist. He called to inform that the results came back from the biopsy as inconclusive. I paused for a moment. I then asked him what that mean for me. He stated that a determination could not be made if I had cancer or not and that I just needed to go and see the surgeon that he was referring me to. I was confused and then became anxious because inconclusive is not telling anything and I really need to know if I have cancer or not. His next response didn't help me either. He stated that it was a possibility that it was cancer but he did not know for sure based on the results of the biopsy. He then told me that Thyroid Cancer is one of the easiest cancers and if anyone had to have cancer that would be the one to have. He then ended the phone call with an apology and suggested that I follow up with the appointment that was made with the surgeon. The call ended. I sat there at my desk for a moment and then I cried. One of the easiest cancers, I thought to myself. I don't want any cancer!!!!!! There is nothing easy about cancer. I just want it to go away if it's there. There has got to be a mistake. Maybe it's not cancer, because it was inconclusive. I came up with as many thoughts about possibilities in my mind. I then gathered my belongings and went on home. It was late and I wanted to keep my thoughts as positive. I didn't believe anything that wasn't there. I kept telling myself that everyone makes mistakes so I will just wait and see what the surgeon has to say. I kept my appointment with the surgeon the following week. I was nervous but looking forward to addressing the problem and getting answers.

I met with the first surgeon that I was referred to by the first Endocrinologist. He had my results in his office in my chart during the surgery consult visit. The surgeon was an older white male. I researched him on the internet prior to my visit to see who I would be dealing with. He had five stars and I felt comfortable with that. The comments were encouraging from previous patients and their experiences. When I arrived at his office, the staff was hospitable. I was taken into an examination room. My blood pressure was elevated and that was mainly because I was nervous and fearful. I was then escorted into another room and moments later, the surgeon came in. He shook my hand rather firmly and introduced himself. He then glanced in my chart and told me that the parathyroid had to be removed. He stated that I had Hyperparathyroidism Disease and this was because of the four, there was one parathyroid that was the culprit and it needed to be removed. He began to explain the process of the surgery. He added that it would be rather quick and I should recover in a very short time. The surgeon then stated that I had another problem. The other problem that he explained was the nodules on my thyroid. He described it as inconclusive which means that there was no determination about if there was cancer present or not. I was confused and began asking questions. My first question was how could the biopsy results be inconclusive, do I have cancer or not? His response to me was that he wasn't sure because it was inconclusive. He then stated to me that he could remove the nodules from my thyroid during the surgery and have them sent to pathology and if it is cancer then he would schedule another surgery and remove the thyroid. I began to cry because I felt that I had to make a decision that I wasn't prepared to make. I understood that my parathyroid had to be removed but I wasn't even prepared to discuss my thyroid. The surgeon then told me that I had some decisions to make. He gave me the option to just have my thyroid removed and take medication to replace the thyroid hormone for the remainder of my life or just remove the nodule off my thyroid and wait and see with the possibility of another surgery. I was afraid and sobbed like a baby. He gave me a box of tissue and waited. I then proceeded to ask him a question. He looked at me and paused while I was leading up to asking him if early menopause is the result of the problems that I was experiencing with my thyroid. I was formulating the question to inquire as to whether or not I had the thyroid problems long before without knowing. During that brief moment I was not formulating my question fast enough and he abruptly stated to me, "Get to the point." I was crying and stopped suddenly. I waited for his answer. His response was, "No." He then told me to think about what I wanted him to do in terms of removing a part of my thyroid where the nodules were present or removing the entire thyroid. I left the examination room and went to another office to schedule my surgery. I left his office with a feeling of being more confused. I couldn't understand why anyone could not tell me if I had cancer. I had even more to think about now. I constantly asked myself if I should have my entire thyroid removed or should I just have a portion of it removed? I wasn't prepared to make that decision and I didn't want to make it. I sat in my car and cried. I felt so uninformed. I didn't have any answers and was even more confused. Then to even think that the surgeon told me to GET TO THE POINT! I was devastated. I was hurting and I needed more from him. I needed him to understand that I had questions. I was afraid and he just dismissed me. I had a surgery date for him to perform my surgery and was so uncertain about what to do. I didn't want to have my thyroid removed if it wasn't cancerous but then I didn't want to have just a portion removed and later learn that I would have to be cut on again. He never said anything about running any additional tests to check for anything else. I prayed and consulted with family, friends and my co-workers. The support was overwhelming. I was definitely experiencing a storm in my life and needed understanding and clarity. Over the next few days I experienced moments of sadness where I cried. I wanted answers but didn't have a clue.

One night I was in the office working past 5pm which I did most days. My co-worker and dear friend Veronica was in the office with me. As I was preparing to pack up and leave she asked me how I was doing. I told her that I was afraid. She asked me if she could pray with me and I agreed. She prayed with me. I thanked her. She then told me to get a second opinion. I told her that I didn't want a second opinion because I didn't want to prolong anything, I just wanted to get this over and done with. She then looked at me and insisted that I get a second opinion. I left the office that evening giving a lot of thought to what she suggested. I then thought about the money. I thought about the co-pays that I would be required to pay. I further thought about waiting for another appointment and prolonging the process. There was one thing that I realized and understood and that was that I had to have surgery and it was necessary because Hyperparathyroidism Disease is a debilitating disease that shuts the body down over time. I allowed a few days to pass and then Veronica asked me again if I decided to schedule that appointment. I decided to do it. I was disappointed with the surgeon's demeanor. I was even more disappointed that the surgeon and the Endocrinologist were not able to tell me if I had cancer. I had a biopsy and no one was able to provide me with a clear answer about my results. I was left feeling confused and in order to make the best possible decision, I needed to get that second opinion. Veronica was right. I knew better but I just didn't want to entertain the thought that there could be a possibility that there was even any form of cancer in my body. I then began to search the internet again for new providers. I also decided to find a new Endocrinologist. I could not place myself in the hands of a surgeon that was not empathetic and rude enough to tell me to get to the point. He was fired!!!! I canceled the surgery and decided to fire the first Endocrinologist. He was nice but couldn't provide me with a definite answer. I had to move on and establish a new relationship with new doctors. I was in control and I needed to be informed. I am my own advocate and I needed to do this for myself. I found my two new doctors. I am so glad that I did. The timing was perfect. I researched them and I was pleased. I made the initial contact and made arrangements to get my medical records sent to their offices. I selected a female surgeon this time as well as a female Endocrinologist. I scheduled appointments with both new doctors within a week of each other.

I met with the new surgeon and she confirmed for me that I had cancer. I was diagnosed with Papillary Thyroid Cancer. I met with the new Endocrinologist and she was very supportive of my decision to select the surgeon of my choice. She offered to provide continuous follow up care immediately following my surgery. My new surgeon scheduled my surgery for the first week in June. It was time to move forward and get all of this over and done with. I was at a point where I had two wonderful physicians that I felt totally comfortable with. They both answered all of my questions and took as much time with me to ensure that I felt clear and comfortable about what was getting ready to happen. I couldn't be happier. I was afraid about the thought of being put to sleep but eventually I knew that I would have the surgery sooner than later. I had to accept the diagnosis and I did. I had a cancer and there was no time for delay. I didn't want to die there was still too much living to do but I realized now more than ever that each and every moment was crucial moving forward. The surgery was scheduled along with some pre-surgery testing. I was ready because it was time.

Deuteronomy 31:6
New International Version (NIV)

6 Be strong and courageous. Do not be afraid or terrified because of them, for the Lord your God goes with you; he will never leave you nor forsake you."

5

THE BIGGEST FIGHT OF MY LIFE

It was Monday June 6th and I had awakened at 3:30am. It was time. I took my shower and said my prayers. I called my parents and my children. I grabbed my packed bag and off to the hospital my husband and I went. I arrived in plenty of time. We had to check in. It was like being at the airport. We discussed my insurance and what I would be responsible after my insurance pays its portion. I was comfortable knowing that I was in good hands and everything was being done in a state of the art facility. The nurse called my name. She told me that she needed me first. I followed her to the back to the area that is called the surgery waiting area. There were many other people waiting for their Anesthesiologist and Surgeon to come and get them for their surgery. I was nervous and afraid. I kept thinking about not waking up. I had so many thoughts going through my mind. The nurse provided me with a hospital gown and had instructed me to change. I sat in the chair and paused. The nurse's back was turned to me as she was entering my vitals into the computer. She turned around and asked me if I was ok, and I told her that I was not. She asked me what was wrong. I broke down and cried. She offered prayer and I gladly accepted. She prayed with me and then left me alone to get changed into the hospital gown. I changed and got on the gurney to wait for the next step. The nurse came back in and made me comfortable and talked to me to ease my fears. The Anesthesiologist and his team came to introduce themselves. The nurse Anesthetist came along and introduced herself to me. She assured me that she would be with me during my surgery and make me most comfortable. The Surgeon Resident Physician that was assigned to assist my surgeon came and introduced himself to me as well. The team was friendly and comforting. Then at last, my surgeon came. She was smiling and bubbly. She greeted me and asked me how I was doing. I told her that I was afraid and she told me that I would be fine and that she would take care of me. She then told me that she would see me in the operating room. The Anesthesiologist then placed medicine in my I.V. to make me feel more relaxed. I began to feel more relax than I was when I first arrived. It was time for battle. It was time for me to be rolled back to the operating room. I was ready. It was time to take cancer down and out!

My surgery was approximately 3.5 hours. I was awakened with my husband right at my side as always. My friend Tashaune was right there as well to see me and wish me well. She made me smile. My mother and daughter came in a few moments later and made my day also. I was still very sleepy and my blood pressure was very high immediately following the surgery. My mother didn't stay long but it was very comforting knowing that she and my daughter were there. Once everyone else left my husband surprised me with a visitor, my dear friend Sharon. I had not seen Sharon in six years but she was right there and stayed most of the evening until my son came.

There were an abundance of prayers and well wishes that were going up everywhere. I received calls, text messages and cards. I didn't fight this battle alone. I had the support of many believers that were in my corner from the very beginning. I remained in the hospital for several hours and ended up going home the following day after my blood pressure had stabilized.

My throat was sore. It was difficult to eat and swallow. I didn't have much of an appetite but had to force myself to eat. I began taking the medication Levothyroxine. My initial dose was 150mcg. Levothyroxine is a replacement for a hormone normally produced by the thyroid gland to regulate the body's energy and metabolism. Levothyroxine is given when the thyroid does not produce enough of this hormone on its own. It treats hypothyroidism (low thyroid hormone). It is also used to treat or prevent goiter (enlarged thyroid gland), which can be caused by hormone imbalances, radiation treatment, surgery, or cancer. I had to take Vitamin D and a Calcium supplement as well. I went from having too much calcium to not having enough calcium.

The nurses were amazing. I had the most pleasant experience. I was so glad that it was over. I woke from the surgery with a hope. I fought the cancer and it was over, at least for now. I couldn't thank God enough that the surgery over and he had brought me through the battle.

It was challenging getting to this point. There were times that I didn't think that I would get there but I did. I made it through by the Grace of God! I was blessed beyond measure. God placed all of the right people in my path at the right time. I needed answers and He allowed me to get the answers even if they were from people that I least expected.

I recovered for about four weeks. The first two weeks following surgery I slept a lot. I drank lots of hot tea. There were times after the surgery that I would talk and then suddenly get tired and have to stop talking. I ate plenty of throat lozenges (cough drops). The lemon flavor was soothing and it helped. I recall a few times when I would be speaking and then lose my voice in the middle of a conversation. As time passed, that happened less and my vocal cords got stronger.

I returned for my post-op appointment with the surgeon. She greeted me with a hug and with a smile she told me that together, "We got the cancer." I had tears in my eyes. I was grateful and humble. She told me that the cancer was contained only on the thyroid. She added that the parathyroid was removed and that was benign (Non-cancerous). She provided other details about my surgery that were very important. The cancer was small about the size of a half of a pinky fingernail. The other areas in my neck were clear and the cancer had not spread to any other area in my body. I was relieved and thankful. Words could not begin to express how humble I felt at that moment. She hugged me and wished me the best moving forward. I had blood work at the cancer center and instructed to follow up with my new Endocrinologist.

I followed up with my new Endocrinologist and had to have more blood work to compare with previous blood work to ensure that my levels were where they were supposed to be since having the thyroidectomy (removal of my thyroid). My energy level had increased. I definitely could feel a difference since having my parathyroid removed. The removal of the parathyroid corrected the Hyperparathyroidism Disease and the removal of the thyroid corrected the cancer. The cancer was gone. I had begun to feel so much better since the parathyroid was removed. I didn't feel exhausted like I did previously and I didn't have the foggy memory or constipation like I did previously. I felt great and it had been a long time since I felt that way. During my appointment with my new Endocrinologist, it was determined that my dosage of Levothyroxine (150 mcg) was too much and my dosage was lowered to 137 mcg. A few weeks later in a follow up visit I was told that I did not have to have the Radioactive Iodine Therapy (RAI) since having my surgery. My test results were low enough at this time but that could change if my test results are ever elevated.

Radioactive iodine therapy, also known as RAI, is used following surgery for certain types of thyroid cancer; specifically, follicular and papillary and may also be useful for some differentiated types. When a patient receives RAI, the doctor administers radioactive iodine to destroy thyroid cells, while not harming cells from other organs. The majority of radioactive iodine, therefore, will be absorbed by any remaining thyroid cells.

James 4:10
New International Version (NIV)

10 Humble yourselves before the Lord, and he will lift you up.

6

A HUMBLING EXPERIENCE

The surgery was over and that experience was one that I don't want to ever experience again. I went through so many emotions. I cried many nights and reached out to many people for prayer and comfort. I am blessed that the many people that I turned to was receptive and comforting. There was never a time when anyone turned me away. I will forever be humbled by this experience. It has impacted my life in a way that will exist within my soul forever.

To say that this is a humbling experience is an understatement. The lens of my eyes will view life differently. The little things that I took for granted such as the ability to tell someone I love you or to do something for myself, has greater meaning to me now than anything materialistic. Materialistic things are items that can be touched, lost, broken, and replaced. To tell someone how you feel and the ability to be mobile and experience moments whether good or bad, are moments that will always be remembered. The things that we remember are the pictures in the mind that the soul rehearses for us from time to time that we refer to as memory. This is a memory that will always be with me and at times it will remind where I was and how I got through this to get where I am today. I understand and I realize that I could not have gotten through this without the Grace of God. My mind allows me to reflect back often and I know that things could have been different. I know that it was only God that brought me through this battle. The battle was not mine, it was his. He placed me in position to fight and appointed several others to experience this battle with me.

I will not live a life in a delayed state of mind. I realize through my experience that putting anything off for tomorrow is no longer an option. Life is so short and I was given another chance to make a difference in my own life. I feel that I had another opportunity to fix any wrongs in my life and forgive those who may have wronged me. I realize now that there is no additional time. It is never too late while my feet are above ground but walking around with the expectation of having extra time is senseless. There is no such thing as extra time. The time that has been given is appointed and every moment of that time counts. It is up to me how I choose to utilize the time allotted.

The moments wasted on anger, worry, defeat, and disappointment is time that can never be replaced.

A cancer diagnosis has given me the chance to make some changes and really examine my time and utilize it wisely. There should never be a day that ends in regrets unless you are waiting for something from someone else to deliver in which you have no control of. When I was told that I had cancer, my life stopped immediately. I was filled with emotions that I could not control and I regurgitated everything hidden in my soul. I couldn't believe that I was diagnosed with cancer. I wanted it to go away and pretended at times that it did not exist. I allowed my mind to suspend certain moments in time so I would not have to relive them again. The one thing that is for certain, anything hidden will surface again and when you are not prepared it's like a volcano with a messy aftermath.

I had to do something about the cancer. I wasn't prepared for the battle until I accepted the fact that I did have cancer. The moment I embraced it, I prepared for the fight and empowered myself emotionally to give it everything that I had left in me to beat it. I recall making phone calls, sending text messages and other notes to close family and friends. I told them about my diagnosis but a part of me wanted their sympathy and their pity. I wanted others to cry with me but although many were sadden, they never allowed me to see their sadness for me. My husband never allowed me to think about the cancer and he made sure that my mind was thinking about positive things. My parents constantly told me to pray as they prayed for me daily. My children always spoke of tackling the cancer and coming out on top. Then there was everyone else who prayed for me and told others to pray for me too. This was all so humbling for me.

Another humbling moment for me was the days and time spent in the cancer center. I observed for myself that cancer is not defined by an age group, ethnicity, gender, or socioeconomic status. I saw everyone at the cancer center. I was sadden and heartbroken while God was humbling me at the same time. I cried when I saw that man that could hardly make it and he appeared to be walking alone, then there was the woman with no hair that seem to push a smile through her frail face while daunting a beautiful scarf adorning her clean head.

I went inside the gift shop that was located within the cancer center and was greeted by two lovely elderly ladies. I walked through and looked at the beautiful scarves, t-shirts, pens, and buttons. Every type of cancer was represented. I was moved to purchase a shirt and a keychain. I also saw wigs and hats for sale too. The money made through purchases at the gift shop goes toward the cancer patients and their guests. It was a moving experience for me, to say the least. I was in awe at how other survivors appeared to have held themselves together in their moment of pain. It was encouraging for me to see other people walk their journey. It gave me hope during my journey. Cancer is an experience. It is one that once you have gone through it; you must pay it forward to others that are going through too. You pay it forward with kind words of encouragement, prayers, support, and love. These are the most important things to a cancer warrior.

2 Corinthians 9:6
New International Version (NIV)

6 Remember this: Whoever sows sparingly will also reap sparingly, and whoever sows generously will also reap generously.

7

THE PRICELESS GIFT

Everyone enjoys receiving gifts. To receive a gift means that someone took time out of their day and placed thought and time into you. I never met anyone who didn't like receiving a gift. I love gifts. I always receive a gift humbly because the person that gave the gift didn't have to give the gift. I was always taught as a child that when someone gives you anything you express your appreciation in the form of a "Thank you" note or card. People don't have to acknowledge you or give a gift. Some people don't have it to give and others have it and chose not to give. Gifts that are materialistic are exciting when they are first received but as time pass so does the excitement and then the gift loses its value.

I received the ultimate gift on the day when I was told by my surgeon during my post op visit that all of the cancer in my body was gone. It was a profound moment for me. I had been given an opportunity to embrace my own life again. It was the priceless gift, the gift of life, a gift from God. It is the only gift that I will ever receive that will forever have the most meaning and will impact my life forever. I am so thankful to God for allowing me to have this chance to really live again.

Living now will be very different than it was before. I had many moments of pause when I had to stop abruptly and reflect. I had time to think about where I was, where I am and where I am going. God has been so good to me. He took me through one of the greatest battles of all time. I never had the courage to fight so fiercely like I did during my recent battle with cancer.

I won't ever take those little things for granted anymore. It is a gift when you can do anything and everything for yourself. It is a gift when you can walk across the sand and extend your feet in the water as the waves rush up and wet your feet. It is a gift when you can pick up a pen and write a note and share something with someone else that will impact their life for a lifetime. It is a gift from me to you who reads this, to share my journey with you and to offer my support and prayers to you and those you love.

I am blessed that I can open my eyes and see the beauty of this world out of the lens of my own. I can walk barefooted in the grass as I place one foot in front of the other. I can inhale and exhale all of the air that I breathe without assistance and support. It is only God that made all of this possible. I have another snapshot at life and another chance to make it right. I never thought that I was doing anything wrong but I always have a chance to do something new and something greater.

Each day that I can wake up and breathe the fresh air and taste my own food and see the beauty in nature that God places before me in the various trees, flowers, plants, and animals, I know that I am blessed. Each day that I can speak a word, whisper a prayer, or put a pen between my fingers then I know that I am blessed. I realize that each day is and will forever be my priceless gift. It is not promised but it is appreciated. The time is short and therefore time should not be wasted but utilized in a manner as if time is soon to run out. This is one gift that I will forever cherish and be eternally grateful for. I share my praises with my family and friends and anyone who I encounter on this journey. I have left people speechless when I share the goodness of God and how He has shown me Mercy in delivering my body and healing me completely of cancer.

Colossians 3:16
New International Version (NIV)

16 Let the message of Christ dwell among you richly as you teach and admonish one another with all wisdom through psalms, hymns, and songs from the Spirit, singing to God with gratitude in your hearts.

8

THANK YOU

I am overwhelmed with thanks and praise that I don't know hardly where to begin. The best way to begin is simply to say, "Thank you." I have to thank everyone together because if I begin to name names then I might forget someone and I certainly don't want to do that. I appreciate all of the prayers, calls, text messages, kind words, cards, and hugs. I am and will forever be humbled by this experience.

When I first learned that I had cancer, it was more like a death sentence. It was devastating and heart wrenching. The only thing I initially thought about was death. I was comforted by so many and I was empowered and encouraged to fight a good fight. My son always says, "The moment a person is born the process of death begins." As much as I wanted to dismiss that thought I was faced with it during my journey on the battlefield.

I thought about the many people who began their battle with cancer and lost. I often think about the people who are still fighting and will continue to fight until they win their battle or ultimately lose to cancer. My heart and prayers are with them and their families.

There is one thing for sure and that is, we are all born to die. Each person has an appointed time and I am so thankful that God gave me an extension through my healing. I am thankful that I have another opportunity to share my story and to help others who are dealing with a battle of cancer. I thank God and give Him all of the glory and praise for comforting me on this scary part of the journey. I don't know what tomorrow holds but I do know that my tomorrow is in God's hands and the ultimate plan is His.

I want to acknowledge my family, friends, and co-workers for the love and support. There were many people that placed my name on the prayer list at their church and that meant so much to me. It was so peaceful to know that there were always an army of believers praying for me. I am just overwhelmed with thanks and I will always be thankful. I will never forget the kindness and love bestowed upon me during this emotional time in my life.

I finally have to thank the Physicians and staff at Duke University Medical Center in Durham, North Carolina and Duke University Cancer Center. They were all phenomenal. I was in the right place at the right time. There are not enough words to express my sincerest thanks. I am so grateful for the exceptional care and support that I received. I will not ever forget this moment in time. Thank you.

Thank you again to everyone. From the bottom of my heart, I thank you very much.

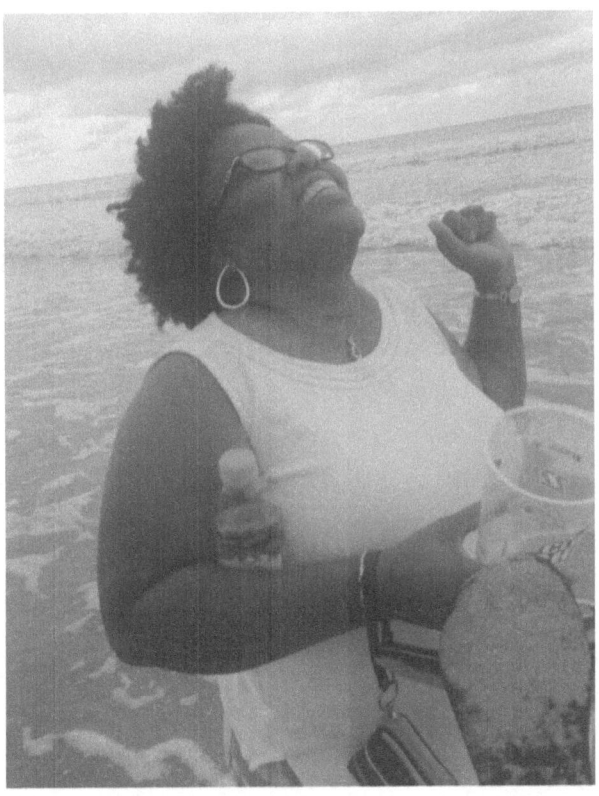

Hebrews 13:13-15
New International Version (NIV)

15 Through Jesus, therefore, let us continually offer to God a sacrifice of praise—the fruit of lips that openly profess his name.

www.ingramcontent.com/pod-product-compliance
Lightning Source LLC
Chambersburg PA
CBHW030536290526
45786CB00004B/1732